GERD DIET
COOKBOOK
FOR SENIORS

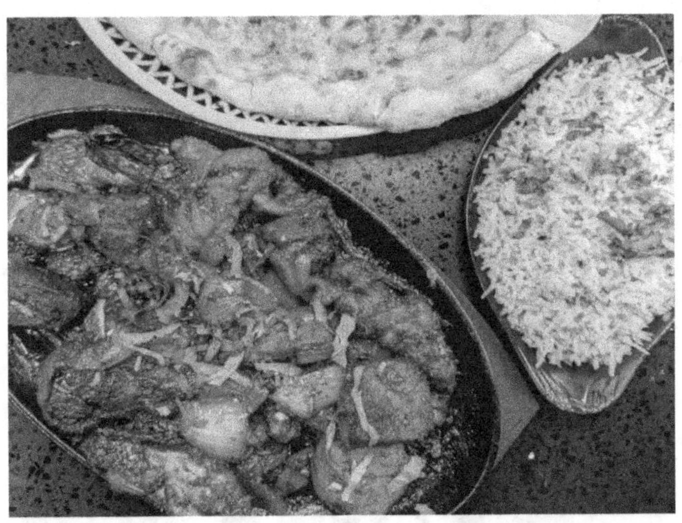

"Nutritious Guide with Easy Recipes for Effective Weight Loss and to Manage Acid Reflux"

Dayna G. Murphy

Copyright © 2024 by Dayna G. Murphy

All rights reserved.

GAIN ACCESS TO OTHER BOOKS BY ME

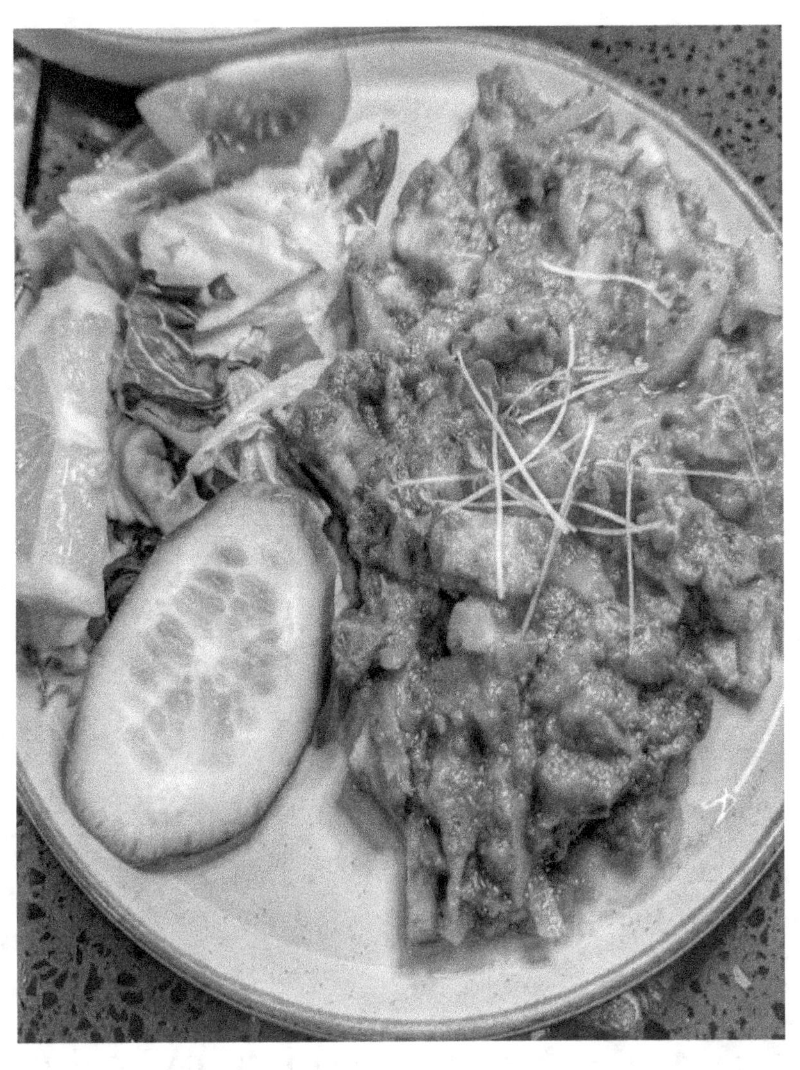

TABLE OF CONTENTS

INTRODUCTION

Welcome to **"GERD Diet Cookbook for Seniors,"** your essential guide to maintaining a healthy and enjoyable lifestyle while managing Gastroesophageal Reflux Disease (GERD). This cookbook is crafted with the well-being of seniors in mind, offering a collection of delicious recipes designed to soothe and nourish, all while adhering to GERD-friendly dietary principles.

Purpose of the Book

In the golden years, health becomes paramount, and GERD, a prevalent digestive condition, can pose challenges to seniors' well-being. This cookbook aims to empower seniors with practical knowledge and delectable recipes tailored to alleviate GERD symptoms. By embracing a GERD-friendly diet, seniors can enjoy their favorite meals without compromising their digestive health.

Importance of a GERD-Friendly Diet for Seniors

Understanding the significance of a GERD-friendly diet is crucial for seniors seeking to enhance their quality of life. GERD, characterized by acid reflux and heartburn, can exacerbate with age, leading to discomfort and potential complications. This cookbook addresses the unique dietary needs of seniors, providing solutions to minimize acid reflux, promote digestion, and foster overall wellness. By making informed choices and embracing the recipes within, seniors can savor delicious meals while actively managing their GERD, ensuring a more vibrant and fulfilling lifestyle.

Understanding GERD (Gastroesophageal Reflux Disease):

GERD, or Gastroesophageal Reflux Disease, is a chronic condition that occurs when stomach acid frequently flows back into the esophagus, the tube connecting the mouth to the stomach. This backflow of acid can irritate the lining of the esophagus, leading to various symptoms and potential complications.

How GERD Affects Seniors:

Seniors are more prone to experiencing GERD due to several factors, including:

1. Weakening of the Lower Esophageal Sphincter (LES):

The LES is a muscular ring that separates the esophagus from the stomach. With age, this muscle may weaken, allowing stomach acid to reflux into the esophagus more easily.

2. Reduced Stomach Function:

Aging can lead to a decrease in stomach acid production and slower digestion. This can contribute to a longer retention of stomach contents, increasing the likelihood of reflux.

3. Hiatal Hernia:

Seniors may be more prone to hiatal hernias, where a portion of the stomach protrudes into the chest cavity, further contributing to acid reflux.

Symptoms of GERD in Seniors:

Common symptoms of GERD in seniors include:

1. Heartburn:

- A burning sensation or discomfort in the chest, often after eating.

2. Regurgitation:

- The sensation of stomach acid backing up into the throat or mouth.

3. Difficulty Swallowing:

- Seniors with GERD may experience difficulty or pain while swallowing.

4. Chronic Cough:

- Persistent coughing, often due to irritation caused by stomach acid.

5. Sore Throat and Hoarseness:

- Irritation of the throat may lead to a persistent sore throat or changes in voice.

Importance of Managing GERD through Diet:

Managing GERD is crucial for seniors to prevent complications and enhance their overall well-being. Diet plays a pivotal role in this management for several reasons:

1. Minimizing Acidic Triggers:

- Certain foods and beverages can trigger acid reflux. A GERD-friendly diet helps seniors identify and avoid these triggers, reducing the frequency and severity of symptoms.

2. Maintaining a Healthy Weight:

- Excess weight can contribute to GERD symptoms. A balanced diet promotes weight management, potentially alleviating the pressure on the stomach and reducing reflux.

3. Promoting Esophageal Healing:

- Some foods have soothing properties that can help heal and protect the esophagus. Including these in the diet can aid in managing GERD symptoms.

4. Preventing Complications:

- Untreated GERD can lead to complications such as esophagitis, Barrett's esophagus, and even an increased risk of esophageal cancer. Managing the condition through diet can help prevent these serious outcomes.

By embracing a GERD-friendly diet, seniors can actively participate in the management of their condition, experiencing relief from symptoms and improving their overall quality of life. This cookbook aims to guide seniors in making informed dietary choices that contribute to their digestive health and well-being.

CHAPTER 1: THE BASICS OF GERD DIET

OVERVIEW OF GERD-FRIENDLY FOODS

Foods Generally Safe for GERD Sufferers:

1. Non-Citrus Fruits:

- Options like bananas, melons, and pears are low in acidity and are less likely to trigger reflux.

2. Vegetables:

- Non-acidic vegetables such as broccoli, carrots, and green beans are typically well-tolerated.

3. Lean Proteins:

- Skinless poultry, fish, lean cuts of beef, and tofu are good protein sources with lower fat content.

4. Whole Grains:

- Oatmeal, brown rice, quinoa, and whole-grain breads are rich in fiber and less likely to cause reflux.

5. Dairy Alternatives:

- Low-fat or fat-free dairy alternatives like almond milk and soy milk may be suitable for those with GERD.

6. Healthy Fats:

- Avocado, olive oil, and nuts contain healthy fats and are less likely to trigger reflux.

7. Herbs and Spices:

- Ginger, basil, and parsley can add flavor without causing excessive acidity.

8. Non-Caffeinated Beverages:

- Water, herbal teas, and certain non-citrus fruit juices are safer options for hydration.

Why Certain Foods Trigger Acid Reflux and Should Be Avoided:

1. High-Fat Foods:

- Fatty foods slow down digestion, causing the stomach to produce more acid. Fried foods, full-fat dairy, and fatty meats should be limited.

2. Citrus Fruits:

- Citrus fruits (oranges, lemons, grapefruits) are acidic and can irritate the esophagus, triggering reflux.

3. Tomatoes and Tomato-Based Products:

- Tomatoes are acidic, and products like tomato sauce can contribute to acid reflux.

4. Chocolate:

- Chocolate contains substances that can relax the lower esophageal sphincter (LES), allowing acid to flow back into the esophagus.

5. Peppermint and Spearmint:

- Mint can relax the LES, potentially leading to reflux. Avoid peppermint and spearmint-flavored foods and candies.

6. Caffeinated Beverages:

- Coffee, tea, and caffeinated sodas can relax the LES and stimulate acid production, exacerbating GERD symptoms.

7. Spicy Foods:

- Spices and spicy foods can irritate the esophagus and trigger acid reflux in some individuals.

8. Carbonated Beverages:

- Carbonated drinks can introduce gas into the digestive system, causing pressure that may lead to reflux.

9. Onions and Garlic:

- Onions and garlic can relax the LES and may cause irritation, contributing to acid reflux.

10. Mint:

- While not directly acidic, mint can relax the LES, potentially leading to reflux. It's advisable to avoid mint-flavored items.

Understanding the reasons behind certain foods triggering acid reflux allows individuals with GERD to make informed dietary choices. This knowledge empowers them to create a balanced and GERD-friendly diet, promoting better symptom management and overall digestive health.

MEAL PLANNING FOR SENIORS:

Tips on Creating Well-Balanced, Portion-Controlled Meals for GERD:

1. Incorporate a Variety of Foods:

- Include a mix of fruits, vegetables, lean proteins, whole grains, and healthy fats in each meal. This ensures a diverse range of nutrients without relying heavily on potentially triggering ingredients.

2. Focus on Lean Proteins:

- Choose lean protein sources such as poultry, fish, tofu, and legumes. These options are less likely to contribute to reflux and provide essential nutrients.

3. Opt for Whole Grains:

- Choose whole grains like brown rice, quinoa, and whole-grain bread to increase fiber intake and promote digestive health.

4. Include Non-Acidic Vegetables:

- Prioritize non-acidic vegetables such as broccoli, carrots, and leafy greens. These are rich in vitamins and minerals without causing excess acidity.

5. Use Healthy Fats in Moderation:

- Incorporate sources of healthy fats like avocado, olive oil, and nuts, but be mindful of portion sizes to avoid overconsumption.

6. Limit High-Fat and Fried Foods:

- Minimize the intake of high-fat and fried foods, as they can contribute to overproduction of stomach acid and exacerbate GERD symptoms.

7. Watch Portion Sizes:

- Be mindful of portion sizes to prevent overeating. Use smaller plates and bowls, and listen to your body's hunger and fullness cues.

8. Chew Thoroughly:

- Chew food slowly and thoroughly. This aids digestion and reduces the likelihood of swallowing excess air, which can contribute to bloating and reflux.

9. Stay Hydrated with Water:

- Drink water throughout the day to stay hydrated. Avoid large amounts of fluid during meals to prevent overfilling the stomach and putting pressure on the LES.

10. Plan Balanced Snacks:

- If snacking between meals, choose GERD-friendly options like fresh fruits, yogurt, or a handful of nuts to maintain energy levels without overloading the digestive system.

Emphasize the Importance of Regular Eating Schedules:

1. Consistent Meal Times:

- Stick to regular meal times to establish a routine for your digestive system. Consistency can help manage GERD symptoms by promoting stable acid production.

2. Avoid Skipping Meals:

- Skipping meals can lead to overeating later in the day. Aim for regular, balanced meals to maintain steady energy levels and support digestive health.

3. Space Out Meals and Snacks:

- Plan meals and snacks with enough time in between to allow for proper digestion. Avoid eating large meals close to bedtime to reduce the risk of nighttime reflux.

4. Create a Meal Schedule:

- Develop a daily meal schedule that aligns with your lifestyle. Having a plan can help you make healthier food choices and maintain portion control.

5. Mindful Eating Practices:

- Practice mindful eating by focusing on your meal, savoring each bite, and paying attention to feelings of fullness. This can prevent overeating and improve digestion.

By incorporating these tips into your daily routine, you can create well-balanced, portion-controlled meals that support digestive health and help manage GERD symptoms effectively. Establishing regular eating schedules further contributes to a healthier and more comfortable lifestyle.

CHAPTER 2: ESSENTIAL INGREDIENTS AND COOKING TECHNIQUES

GERD-FRIENDLY INGREDIENTS:

Staple Ingredients Suitable for GERD Diets:

1. Lean Proteins:

- Chicken breast
- Turkey
- Fish (salmon, trout, cod)
- Tofu
- Lean cuts of beef
- or pork

2. Non-Acidic Vegetables:

- Broccoli
- Carrots
- Green beans
- Spinach

- Kale

3. Whole Grains:

- Brown rice
- Quinoa
- Oats
- Whole-grain bread
- Barley

4. Healthy Fats:

- Avocado
- Olive oil
- Flaxseeds
- Chia seeds
- Almonds

5. Non-Citrus Fruits:

- Bananas
- Melons (cantaloupe, honeydew)
- Apples
- Pears
- Berries (strawberries, blueberries)

6. Dairy Alternatives:

- Almond milk

- Soy milk
- Oat milk
- Low-fat or fat-free yogurt

7. Herbs and Spices:

- Ginger
- Basil
- Parsley
- Cilantro
- Dill

8. Whole Foods:

- Beans (black beans, lentils)
- Sweet potatoes
- Cauliflower
- Quinoa
- Chia seeds

9. Non-Citrus Fruit Juices:

- Apple juice
- Pear juice
- Watermelon juice

10. Non-Caffeinated Beverages:

- Water
- Herbal teas (chamomile, ginger, licorice)

- Decaffeinated coffee

Substitutions for Common Trigger Ingredients:

1. Replace Citrus Fruits with Non-Acidic Options:

- Substitute oranges and grapefruits with apples, pears, or berries for a less acidic alternative.

2. Choose Low-Fat Dairy Alternatives:

- Opt for almond milk, soy milk, or oat milk instead of full-fat dairy to reduce fat content.

3. Herb and Spice Alternatives:

- Use ginger, basil, and parsley for flavor instead of trigger-inducing spices like mint and chili.

4. Lean Protein Choices:

- Choose lean proteins like chicken, turkey, and fish over higher fat options like red meat.

5. Whole Grain Substitutes:

- Swap white bread and rice with whole-grain alternatives like brown rice and whole-grain bread.

6. Healthy Fats Instead of Saturated Fats:

- Replace saturated fats with healthier options like avocados, olive oil, and nuts.

7. Non-Citrus Fruit Juices as Alternatives:

- Choose apple or pear juice instead of orange or grapefruit juice for a less acidic option.

8. Non-Caffeinated Beverage Options:

- Opt for herbal teas or decaffeinated coffee instead of regular coffee and caffeinated sodas.

9. Careful with High-Fat Snacks:

- Instead of fried and high-fat snacks, choose nuts, seeds, or whole fruits for healthier options.

10. Mindful Cooking Techniques:

- Grilling, baking, or steaming food instead of frying can reduce fat content and make meals more GERD-friendly.

These staple ingredients and substitutions can form the basis of a nutritious and GERD-friendly diet. By incorporating these choices into your meals, you can enjoy a diverse range of flavors while minimizing the risk of triggering acid reflux.

COOKING TECHNIQUES FOR SENIORS:

Simplified Cooking Methods for Seniors:

1. Grilling:

- Grilling is a straightforward method that imparts a delicious flavor to meats and vegetables. Season, place on the grill, and cook until done.

2. One-Pan Roasting:

- Roasting vegetables and lean proteins on a single pan simplifies cleanup. Toss ingredients with olive oil and herbs, then roast in the oven.

3. Steaming:

- Steaming is an easy and gentle method. Place vegetables or fish in a steamer basket over boiling water, cover, and cook until tender.

4. Slow Cooking:

- Slow cookers are perfect for hands-off cooking. Combine ingredients in the morning, and by evening, you'll have a flavorful and tender meal.

5. Simple Stir-Frying:

- Stir-frying involves quickly cooking small pieces of vegetables and proteins in a pan. Use minimal oil and choose colorful veggies for a nutritious dish.

6. Microwaving:

- Microwaving is quick and efficient. Steam vegetables in the microwave or reheat leftovers for an easy meal.

7. No-Cook Meals:

- Assemble salads, wraps, or sandwiches using pre-cut vegetables, canned beans, and lean proteins for a hassle-free meal.

8. Blending:

- Smoothies are a simple way to combine fruits, vegetables, and yogurt for a nutritious and easily digestible meal or snack.

Easy-to-Follow Recipes with Minimal Preparation Steps:

1. Grilled Chicken Salad:

- Season chicken breasts with herbs and grill until cooked through. Toss with pre-washed salad greens, cherry tomatoes, and a light vinaigrette.

2. Sheet Pan Veggie Bake:

- Coat a mix of vegetables (sweet potatoes, bell peppers, zucchini) with olive oil and roast on a sheet pan alongside seasoned chicken thighs for a simple one-pan meal.

3. Steamed Salmon with Lemon:

- Place salmon fillets in a steamer basket, sprinkle with lemon juice and dill, and steam until the fish is flaky.

4. Slow Cooker Vegetable Soup:

- Combine pre-cut vegetables, broth, and lean protein in a slow cooker. Set it in the morning, and return to a comforting, ready-to-eat soup.

5. Simple Stir-Fried Quinoa:

- Stir-fry cooked quinoa with colorful vegetables, tofu or shrimp, and a splash of low-sodium soy sauce for a quick and nutritious dish.

6. Microwaveable Veggie Omelet:

- Whisk eggs, add diced vegetables, and microwave for a quick omelet. Serve with whole-grain toast for a balanced meal.

7. No-Cook Greek Salad Wrap:

- Fill a whole-grain wrap with pre-cut cucumber, cherry tomatoes, feta cheese, and rotisserie chicken. Drizzle with olive oil for a quick, no-cook meal.

8. Berry Smoothie Bowl:

- Blend mixed berries, yogurt, and a banana. Top with granola and nuts for a satisfying and easily prepared smoothie bowl.

These simplified cooking methods and easy-to-follow recipes minimize preparation steps, making it convenient for seniors to enjoy nutritious and flavorful meals without the stress of complicated cooking processes.

CHAPTER 3: BREAKFASTS TO START THE DAY RIGHT

MORNING SMOOTHIES AND DRINKS

1. Banana Berry Bliss:

Ingredients:

- 1 ripe banana
- 1/2 cup mixed berries (strawberries, blueberries, raspberries)
- 1/2 cup non-citrus fruit juice (apple or pear)
- 1/2 cup plain Greek yogurt
- 1 tablespoon chia seeds

Instructions:

- Blend all ingredients until smooth. Adjust consistency with water if needed. Enjoy this refreshing, non-acidic smoothie.

2. Melon Mint Cooler:

Ingredients:

- 1 cup honeydew or cantaloupe, cubed
- 1/2 cup cucumber, peeled and diced

- 1/2 cup almond milk

- Fresh mint leaves (to taste)

- Ice cubes

Instructions:

- Blend melon, cucumber, almond milk, and mint until smooth. Add ice cubes and blend again for a cooling, soothing smoothie.

3. Pineapple Paradise:

Ingredients:

- 1 cup fresh pineapple, diced

- 1/2 cup coconut water

- 1/2 cup non-citrus fruit (e.g., apple) juice

- 1/2 cup coconut milk (unsweetened)

- 1 tablespoon ground flaxseeds

Instructions:

- Blend pineapple, coconut water, fruit juice, coconut milk, and flaxseeds until creamy. Sip on this tropical delight without the acidity.

ALTERNATIVES TO ACIDIC OR TRIGGER-RICH BREAKFAST OPTIONS:

1. Oatmeal with Banana and Almond Butter:

- Cook old-fashioned oats with water or non-citrus fruit juice. Top with sliced bananas and a dollop of almond butter for a hearty, GERD-friendly breakfast.

2. Greek Yogurt Parfait:

- Layer non-fat Greek yogurt with granola, sliced strawberries, and a drizzle of honey for a satisfying and protein-rich breakfast without triggering acidity.

3. Egg White Vegetable Scramble:

- Cook egg whites with colorful vegetables (bell peppers, spinach, tomatoes) using minimal oil. Season with herbs and serve with whole-grain toast for a nutritious, low-acid breakfast.

4. Chia Pudding with Berries:

- Mix chia seeds with almond milk and let it sit overnight. Top with fresh berries in the morning for a fiber-rich, no-cook breakfast option.

5. Smoothie Bowl with Greens:

- Blend spinach, banana, non-citrus fruits, and almond milk. Pour into a bowl and top with granola, nuts, and seeds for a nutrient-packed breakfast without triggering reflux.

6. Whole-Grain Toast with Avocado:

- Spread mashed avocado on whole-grain toast. Sprinkle with a pinch of salt and pepper for a simple, satisfying breakfast that's gentle on the stomach.

7. Baked Sweet Potato with Cinnamon:

- Bake a sweet potato and sprinkle with cinnamon. This provides a nutrient-rich and filling breakfast option with minimal preparation.

NUTRIENT-RICH BREAKFAST DISHES:

1. Banana Oatmeal Porridge:

Ingredients:

- 1/2 cup old-fashioned oats
- 1 cup water or non-citrus fruit juice
- 1 ripe banana, mashed
- 1 tablespoon almond butter
- Cinnamon for flavor

Instructions:

- Cook oats with water or fruit juice until creamy.
- Stir in mashed banana and almond butter.
- Sprinkle with cinnamon.

Enjoy this comforting and easily digestible porridge.

2. Yogurt and Berry Parfait:

Ingredients:

- 1 cup non-fat Greek yogurt
- 1/2 cup mixed berries (blueberries, raspberries, strawberries)
- 2 tablespoons granola
- Drizzle of honey

Instructions:

- Layer Greek yogurt with berries in a glass or bowl.
- Sprinkle granola on top and drizzle with honey.

A light and refreshing parfait that's gentle on the stomach.

3. Scrambled Tofu with Spinach:

Ingredients:

- 1/2 cup firm tofu, crumbled
- Handful of fresh spinach
- 1 teaspoon olive oil
- Salt and pepper to taste

Instructions:

- Sauté crumbled tofu in olive oil until lightly browned.
- Add fresh spinach and cook until wilted.

- Season with salt and pepper.

A protein-rich and stomach-friendly alternative to traditional scrambled eggs.

4. Papaya and Cottage Cheese Bowl:

Ingredients:

- 1 cup ripe papaya, diced
- 1/2 cup low-fat cottage cheese
- 1 tablespoon chopped mint
- 1 teaspoon honey

Instructions:

- Mix diced papaya and cottage cheese in a bowl.
- Sprinkle with chopped mint and drizzle with honey.

A simple and digestive-friendly tropical breakfast.

5. Chia Seed Pudding with Almond Milk:

Ingredients:

- 3 tablespoons chia seeds
- 1 cup unsweetened almond milk

- 1/2 teaspoon vanilla extract
- Fresh berries for topping

Instructions:

- Combine chia seeds, almond milk, and vanilla extract. Stir well.
- Refrigerate overnight.
- Top with fresh berries before serving.

A nutrient-packed and easy-to-digest pudding.

6. Gingered Carrot Smoothie:

Ingredients:

- 1 cup carrots, chopped
- 1/2 cup non-citrus fruit juice (e.g., apple)
- 1/2 cup coconut water
- 1/2 teaspoon fresh ginger, grated
- Ice cubes

Instructions:

- Blend chopped carrots, fruit juice, coconut water, and ginger until smooth.
- Add ice cubes and blend again.

A soothing and stomach-friendly smoothie.

CHAPTER 4: LIGHT LUNCHES AND SNACKS

GERD-FRIENDLY LOW-ACID SANDWICHES AND WRAPS

1. Turkey and Avocado Wrap:

Ingredients:

- Whole-grain or gluten-free wrap
- Sliced turkey breast
- Avocado slices
- Leafy greens (e.g., spinach or arugula)
- Dijon mustard (optional)

Instructions:

- Lay the wrap flat and layer turkey, avocado, and greens.
- Add a drizzle of Dijon mustard if desired.
- Roll the wrap tightly and cut in half.

A satisfying and reflux-friendly option.

2. Chicken and Veggie Pita Pocket:

Ingredients:

- Whole wheat or spelt pita pocket
- Grilled chicken strips
- Sliced cucumber
- Cherry tomatoes, halved
- Greek yogurt dressing

Instructions:

- Stuff the pita pocket with grilled chicken, cucumber, and cherry tomatoes.
- Drizzle with Greek yogurt dressing.

A light and flavorful pita pocket that's easy on the stomach.

3. Egg Salad Lettuce Wraps:

Ingredients:

- Romaine lettuce leaves
- Hard-boiled eggs, chopped
- Greek yogurt
- Dill, chopped
- Salt and pepper to taste

Instructions:

- Mix chopped hard-boiled eggs with Greek yogurt, dill, salt, and pepper.

- Spoon the egg salad into romaine lettuce leaves.

A low-carb, protein-rich alternative to traditional sandwiches.

4. Veggie Hummus Wrap:

Ingredients:

- Spinach or whole-grain wrap
- Hummus
- Sliced bell peppers
- Cucumber, thinly sliced
- Shredded carrots

Instructions:

- Spread a layer of hummus on the wrap.
- Add sliced bell peppers, cucumber, and shredded carrots.
- Roll up the wrap and slice into smaller portions.

A plant-based and reflux-friendly option.

ALTERNATIVES TO HEAVY, TRIGGER-INDUCING SNACKS:

1. Baked Sweet Potato Fries:

- Slice sweet potatoes into fries, toss with a bit of olive oil, and bake until golden. A nutritious alternative to greasy snacks.

2. Greek Yogurt with Berries:

- Enjoy a bowl of non-fat Greek yogurt with fresh berries. Rich in protein and antioxidants without the acidity of other snacks.

3. Rice Cake with Almond Butter:

- Spread almond butter on a rice cake for a satisfying and easy-to-digest snack.

4. Vegetable Sticks with Hummus:

- Dip sliced cucumber, bell pepper, and carrot sticks into hummus for a crunchy and stomach-friendly snack.

5. Baked Apple Slices with Cinnamon:

- Slice apples, sprinkle with cinnamon, and bake until tender. A sweet treat without triggering acidity.

6. Mixed Nuts and Seeds:

- Create a mix of almonds, walnuts, and pumpkin seeds for a nutrient-dense snack. Avoid salted varieties for better digestion.

These sandwich and snack ideas focus on GERD-friendly ingredients, emphasizing lean proteins, fresh vegetables, and whole grains while steering clear of trigger-inducing components. Incorporate these options for a variety of satisfying and reflux-friendly meals.

SNACK IDEAS FOR SENIORS

1. Yogurt Parfait:

- Non-fat Greek yogurt layered with fresh berries and a sprinkle of granola. This snack provides protein, probiotics, and antioxidants without excess acidity.

2. Rice Cake with Cottage Cheese:

- A rice cake topped with low-fat cottage cheese and a drizzle of honey. This combination offers a mix of protein and carbohydrates.

3. Hummus and Veggie Sticks:

- Fresh cucumber, bell pepper, and carrot sticks paired with hummus for a satisfying and nutrient-rich snack that's easy to digest.

4. Baked Sweet Potato Chips:

- Thinly slice sweet potatoes, toss with a touch of olive oil, and bake until crisp. A crunchy and wholesome alternative to traditional chips.

5. Almond Butter and Banana:

- Spread almond butter on banana slices for a nutritious, potassium-rich snack that provides healthy fats and protein.

6. Cottage Cheese with Pineapple:

- Low-fat cottage cheese paired with fresh pineapple chunks. This snack combines protein with the digestive benefits of pineapple enzymes.

7. Chia Seed Pudding:

- Mix chia seeds with almond milk, add a touch of vanilla extract, and refrigerate until it thickens. Top with a few berries for a fiber-rich and satisfying snack.

8. Oat and Nut Energy Balls:

- Combine oats, nuts (like almonds or walnuts), honey, and a dash of cinnamon. Form into small energy balls for a quick, portable snack.

9. Hard-Boiled Eggs with Whole-Grain Crackers:

- Pair hard-boiled eggs with whole-grain crackers for a balanced snack that provides protein and complex carbohydrates.

10. Fresh Fruit Salad:

- A mix of diced melons, berries, and grapes for a refreshing and vitamin-packed snack without excessive acidity.

11. Cherry Tomatoes with Mozzarella:

- Enjoy cherry tomatoes paired with small mozzarella balls or cubes for a light and flavorful snack.

12. Trail Mix with Nuts and Dried Fruit:

- Create a homemade trail mix with unsalted nuts, seeds, and small portions of dried fruits for a satisfying and portable option.

Remember to monitor portion sizes and pay attention to how your body responds to different snacks. These options focus on providing nutrients, fiber, and energy without triggering GERD symptoms.

CHAPTER 5: NOURISHING DINNERS

LEAN PROTEINS AND VEGETABLES:

1. Grilled Lemon Herb Chicken with Roasted Vegetables

Ingredients:

- 2 boneless, skinless chicken breasts
- 1 lemon (zested and juiced)
- 2 tablespoons olive oil
- 2 cloves garlic, minced
- 1 teaspoon dried oregano
- 1 teaspoon dried thyme
- Salt and pepper to taste

For Roasted Vegetables:

- 2 cups mixed non-acidic vegetables (zucchini, bell peppers, cherry tomatoes, carrots)
- 1 tablespoon olive oil
- Salt and pepper to taste

Instructions:

- In a bowl, combine lemon zest, lemon juice, olive oil, minced garlic, dried oregano, dried thyme, salt, and pepper to create the marinade.
- Place chicken breasts in a zip-top bag, pour half of the marinade over them, seal the bag, and marinate in the refrigerator for at least 30 minutes.
- Preheat the grill. Grill the chicken breasts until cooked through, about 6-8 minutes per side.
- While the chicken is grilling, toss the mixed vegetables with olive oil, salt, and pepper. Roast in the oven at 400°F (200°C) for 15-20 minutes or until tender.
- Serve grilled chicken over a bed of roasted vegetables, drizzle with the remaining marinade, and garnish with fresh herbs if desired.

2. Baked Salmon with Quinoa and Steamed Broccoli

Ingredients:

- 2 salmon fillets

- 1 tablespoon Dijon mustard

- 1 tablespoon honey

- 1 teaspoon soy sauce

- 1 cup quinoa, cooked

- 2 cups broccoli florets

- Lemon wedges for serving

- Fresh parsley for garnish

Instructions:

- Preheat the oven to 375°F (190°C).

- In a small bowl, mix Dijon mustard, honey, and soy sauce to create a glaze for the salmon.

- Place salmon fillets on a baking sheet lined with parchment paper. Brush the glaze over the salmon.

- Bake in the preheated oven for 12-15 minutes or until the salmon flakes easily with a fork.

- While the salmon is baking, steam the broccoli until tender-crisp.

- Serve baked salmon over a bed of cooked quinoa, with steamed broccoli on the side.

- Garnish with fresh parsley and serve with lemon wedges.

MINDFUL EATING TIPS:

1. Take smaller bites and chew thoroughly to aid digestion.

2. Put your fork down between bites and savor the flavors.

3. Pay attention to hunger and fullness cues to avoid overeating.

4. Create a calm eating environment, free from distractions.

These recipes offer a balance of lean proteins and non-acidic vegetables, promoting mindful eating and portion control for a satisfying and GERD-friendly dinner.

ONE-POT MEALS FOR CONVENIENCE

1. One-Pan Baked Lemon Garlic Chicken with Vegetables

Ingredients:

- 2 boneless, skinless chicken breasts
- 1 lemon, thinly sliced
- 3 cloves garlic, minced

- 1 tablespoon olive oil

- 1 teaspoon dried thyme

- Salt and pepper to taste

- 2 cups mixed non-acidic vegetables (broccoli, carrots, bell peppers)

Instructions:

- Preheat the oven to 400°F (200°C).

- Place chicken breasts in the center of a baking sheet.

- Surround the chicken with sliced lemon and mixed vegetables.

- Drizzle olive oil over the chicken and vegetables. Sprinkle minced garlic, dried thyme, salt, and pepper.

- Bake in the preheated oven for 20-25 minutes or until the chicken is cooked through and the vegetables are tender.

- Serve directly from the baking sheet. Enjoy a flavorful meal with minimal cleanup.

2. Quick and Easy Veggie Stir-Fry

Ingredients:

- 1 cup mixed non-acidic vegetables (snap peas, bell peppers, carrots)
- 1 cup tofu, diced
- 2 tablespoons low-sodium soy sauce
- 1 tablespoon sesame oil
- 1 teaspoon ginger, grated
- 2 cups cooked brown rice

Instructions:

- Heat sesame oil in a non-stick skillet over medium-high heat.
- Add diced tofu and stir-fry until golden brown.
- Add mixed vegetables and grated ginger. Stir-fry for an additional 3-5 minutes until vegetables are tender-crisp.
- Pour in low-sodium soy sauce and toss to coat evenly.
- Serve the stir-fried tofu and vegetables over cooked brown rice.
- Enjoy this quick and nutritious stir-fry with minimal cleanup.

CLEANUP TIPS FOR SENIORS:

1. Use non-stick cookware to reduce the need for excessive oil and make cleaning easier.

2. Line baking sheets with parchment paper for quick cleanup after baking.

3. Consider using disposable or reusable oven-safe liners to minimize mess.

4. Keep a small trash bin or bag nearby for convenient disposal of vegetable scraps and packaging.

These recipes are designed to be simple, require minimal cleanup, and offer a tasty and balanced meal for seniors.

CHAPTER 6: DESSERTS AND TREATS

GERD-FRIENDLY DESSERTS:

1. Vanilla Chia Pudding:

Ingredients:

- 2 tablespoons chia seeds
- 1 cup almond milk
- 1 teaspoon vanilla extract
- 1 tablespoon honey or maple syrup

Instructions:

1. Mix chia seeds, almond milk, vanilla extract, and sweetener in a jar.

2. Stir well, cover, and refrigerate overnight.

3. Serve chilled, optionally topped with fresh berries or sliced banana.

Alternatives:

1. Use almond or coconut milk instead of dairy.

2. Choose honey or maple syrup as a sweetener over citrus-based sweeteners.

2. Baked Pear with Cinnamon:

Ingredients:

- 2 ripe pears, halved and cored
- 1 tablespoon melted coconut oil
- 1 teaspoon ground cinnamon
- 1 tablespoon chopped nuts (almonds, walnuts)

Instructions:

1. Preheat the oven to 375°F (190°C).

2. Place pear halves in a baking dish.

3. Brush with melted coconut oil and sprinkle with cinnamon.

4. Bake for 25-30 minutes or until pears are tender.

5. Top with chopped nuts before serving.

Alternatives:

1. Coconut oil can be used instead of butter.

2. Opt for non-acidic nuts like almonds or walnuts.

3. Chocolate Avocado Mousse:

Ingredients:

- 2 ripe avocados
- 1/4 cup unsweetened cocoa powder

- 1/4 cup honey or agave syrup
- 1 teaspoon vanilla extract

Instructions:

1. Blend avocados, cocoa powder, honey, and vanilla extract until smooth.

2. Chill in the refrigerator for at least 1 hour.

3. Serve in small bowls, optionally topped with a dollop of whipped cream.

Alternatives:

1. Use honey or agave syrup instead of citrus-based sweeteners.

2. Opt for non-dairy whipped cream if desired.

4. Coconut Rice Pudding:

Ingredients:

- 1/2 cup Arborio rice
- 2 cups coconut milk
- 1/4 cup coconut sugar
- 1 teaspoon vanilla extract
- Ground cinnamon for garnish

Instructions:

1. Combine rice, coconut milk, coconut sugar, and vanilla extract in a saucepan.

2. Cook over medium heat until rice is tender and mixture thickens.

3. Chill and serve topped with a sprinkle of ground cinnamon.

Alternatives:

1. Use coconut sugar as a non-acidic sweetener.

2. Consider adding toasted coconut for texture.

5. Almond Flour Banana Muffins:

Ingredients:

- 2 ripe bananas, mashed
- 2 cups almond flour
- 1/4 cup coconut oil, melted
- 1/4 cup honey
- 2 large eggs
- 1 teaspoon vanilla extract
- 1/2 teaspoon baking soda
- A pinch of salt

Instructions:

1. Preheat the oven to 350°F (175°C). Line a muffin tin with paper liners.

2. In a bowl, mix mashed bananas, almond flour, melted coconut oil, honey, eggs, vanilla extract, baking soda, and salt.

3. Spoon the batter into muffin cups and bake for 18-20 minutes or until a toothpick comes out clean.

Alternatives:

1. Use honey as a non-acidic sweetener.
2. Opt for almond flour instead of acidic refined flours.

6. Pumpkin Spice Oatmeal Cookies:

Ingredients:

- 1 cup rolled oats
- 1/2 cup pumpkin puree
- 1/4 cup coconut oil, melted
- 1/4 cup maple syrup
- 1 teaspoon pumpkin spice
- 1/2 teaspoon vanilla extract

Instructions:

1. Preheat the oven to 350°F (175°C). Line a baking sheet with parchment paper.

2. In a bowl, mix oats, pumpkin puree, melted coconut oil, maple syrup, pumpkin spice, and vanilla extract.

3. Drop spoonfuls onto the baking sheet and bake for 10-12 minutes.

Alternatives:

1.   Use maple syrup as a non-acidic sweetener.

2.   Choose pumpkin spice over citrus-based spices.

7. Coconut Flour Berry Muffins:

Ingredients:

- 1/2 cup coconut flour
- 1/4 cup coconut oil, melted
- 1/4 cup honey
- 4 eggs
- 1/2 teaspoon baking soda
- 1/4 teaspoon salt
- 1 cup mixed berries (blueberries, raspberries)

Instructions:

1. Preheat the oven to 350°F (175°C). Line a muffin tin with paper liners.

2. In a bowl, whisk together coconut flour, melted coconut oil, honey, eggs, baking soda, and salt.

3. Gently fold in mixed berries.

4. Spoon the batter into muffin cups and bake for 20-25 minutes.

Alternatives:

- Use honey as a non-acidic sweetener.
- Opt for coconut flour, a lower-acid alternative.

8. Non-Dairy Vanilla Panna Cotta:

Ingredients:

- 2 cups coconut milk
- 1/4 cup honey or maple syrup
- 1 tablespoon agar-agar powder (plant-based gelatin)
- 1 teaspoon vanilla extract

Instructions:

1. In a saucepan, heat coconut milk, honey or maple syrup, and agar-agar over medium heat.

2. Bring to a simmer, stirring continuously until agar-agar dissolves.

3. Remove from heat, stir in vanilla extract, and pour into ramekins.

4. Chill in the refrigerator until set.

Alternatives:

1. Use honey or maple syrup as a non-acidic sweetener.

2. Opt for coconut milk for a non-dairy alternative.

9. Baked Almond Flour Donuts:

Ingredients:

- 1 cup almond flour
- 1/4 cup coconut sugar
- 1/4 cup coconut oil, melted
- 2 large eggs
- 1/2 teaspoon baking powder
- 1/2 teaspoon vanilla extract

Instructions:

1. Preheat the oven to 350°F (175°C). Grease a donut pan.

2. In a bowl, mix almond flour, coconut sugar, melted coconut oil, eggs, baking powder, and vanilla extract.

3. Spoon the batter into the donut pan and bake for 12-15 minutes.

Alternatives:

1. Use coconut sugar as a non-acidic sweetener.

2. Opt for almond flour instead of acidic refined flours.

10. Cinnamon Baked Pears with Almond Crumble:

Ingredients:

- 4 ripe pears, halved and cored
- 1/4 cup almond flour
- 2 tablespoons coconut oil, melted
- 2 tablespoons chopped almonds
- 1 teaspoon ground cinnamon
- 1 tablespoon honey

Instructions:

1. Preheat the oven to 375°F (190°C).

2. Place pear halves in a baking dish.

3. In a bowl, mix almond flour, melted coconut oil, chopped almonds, ground cinnamon, and honey.

4. Spoon the mixture onto each pear half.

5. Bake for 20-25 minutes or until pears are tender.

Alternatives:

1. Use honey as a non-acidic sweetener.

2. Opt for almond flour instead of acidic refined flours.

These dessert recipes are designed to minimize acidity and provide delicious alternatives to traditional treats. Adjustments can be made based on personal preferences and sensitivities. Enjoy these sweet treats without triggering GERD symptoms!

CHAPTER 7: MEAL PLANS AND TIPS FOR SPECIAL OCCASIONS

Weekly Meal Plans:

DAY 1:

Breakfast:

- Greek Yogurt Parfait with Mixed Berries and Granola

Lunch:

- Turkey and Avocado Wrap with a Side of Sliced Cucumbers

Dinner:

- Grilled Lemon Herb Chicken with Roasted Vegetables (zucchini, carrots, bell peppers)

Snack:

- Almonds and a Small Apple

Grocery Shopping Tips:

Buy non-fat Greek yogurt, mixed berries, granola, turkey breast, whole-grain wraps, avocados, fresh vegetables for roasting, almonds, and apples.

DAY 2:

Breakfast:

- Oatmeal with Banana Slices and Almond Butter

Lunch:

- Egg Salad Lettuce Wraps with Cherry Tomatoes on the Side

Dinner:

- Baked Salmon with Quinoa and Steamed Broccoli

Snack:

- Carrot Sticks with Hummus

Grocery Shopping Tips:

Purchase oats, bananas, almond butter, eggs, lettuce, cherry tomatoes, salmon fillets, quinoa, and broccoli.

DAY 3:

Breakfast:

- Banana-Oat Cookies (from Day 5 recipe)

Lunch:

- Veggie Hummus Wrap with Sliced Bell Peppers

Dinner:

- Coconut Rice Pudding with Sliced Mango

Snack:

- Greek Yogurt with a Drizzle of Honey

Grocery Shopping Tips:

Add bananas, oats, almond flour, hummus, bell peppers, coconut milk, coconut sugar, mango, and non-fat Greek yogurt to your shopping list.

DAY 4:

Breakfast:

- Chia Seed Pudding with Fresh Berries

Lunch:

- Chicken and Veggie Pita Pocket with Greek Yogurt Dressing

Dinner:

- Gingered Carrot Smoothie with a Side of Mixed Nuts

Snack:

- Sliced Pineapple with Cottage Cheese

Grocery Shopping Tips:

Grab chia seeds, mixed berries, chicken breast, whole wheat pita, cucumber, cherry tomatoes, ginger, carrots, almond milk, and cottage cheese.

DAY 5:
Breakfast:

- Vanilla Chia Pudding (from Day 1 recipe)

Lunch:

- Spinach and Feta Salad with Grilled Shrimp

Dinner:

- Quinoa and Vegetable Stir-Fry with Tofu

Snack:

- Baked Apple Slices with Cinnamon

Grocery Shopping Tips:

Pick up chia seeds, almond milk, shrimp, spinach, feta cheese, quinoa, mixed vegetables, and tofu.

DAY 6:
Breakfast:

- Pumpkin Spice Oatmeal Cookies (from Day 5 recipe)

Lunch:

- Tuna Salad Lettuce Wraps with Sliced Cucumbers

Dinner:

- Baked Sweet Potato with Cinnamon and Grilled Chicken

Snack:

- Mixed Nuts and Seeds

Grocery Shopping Tips:

Buy pumpkin spice, canned tuna, lettuce, cucumbers, sweet potatoes, and grilled chicken.

DAY 7:

Breakfast:

- Coconut Flour Berry Muffins (from Day 5 recipe)

Lunch:

- Caprese Salad with Whole-Grain Toast

Dinner:

- Turkey Meatballs with Zucchini Noodles and Marinara Sauce

Snack:

- Fresh Fruit Salad

Grocery Shopping Tips:

Grab coconut flour, mixed berries, mozzarella, tomatoes, basil, whole-grain bread, ground turkey, zucchini, and marinara sauce.

Additional Grocery Shopping Tips for a GERD-Friendly Diet:

1. Choose lean proteins: Opt for skinless poultry, fish, lean cuts of meat, and plant-based protein sources like tofu and legumes.

2. Select whole grains: Purchase whole grains such as quinoa, brown rice, and whole-grain bread to provide fiber and nutrients.

3. Include non-acidic fruits and vegetables: Stock up on bananas, melons, berries, carrots, spinach, and other non-acidic options.

4. Dairy alternatives: Consider non-dairy options like almond or coconut milk and non-fat Greek yogurt.

5. Healthy fats: Choose olive oil, coconut oil, and avocados for cooking and dressing.

6. Herbs and spices: Add flavor with herbs like basil, mint, and oregano, and use spices like cinnamon and ginger.

7. Low-acid sweeteners: Opt for honey, maple syrup, or coconut sugar instead of citrus-based sweeteners.

Eating Out and Socializing:

Making healthy choices when dining out can be challenging, but it's possible to enjoy meals while managing GERD symptoms. Here are some tips for making mindful choices when eating out and managing GERD during social events:

1. Choose GERD-Friendly Restaurants:

- **Look for Options with Grilled Proteins:** Choose restaurants that offer grilled or baked proteins like chicken, fish, or lean cuts of meat. Avoid fried or heavily sauced dishes.

- **Opt for Whole Grains:** Choose dishes that include whole grains such as brown rice, quinoa, or whole wheat pasta.

2. Mindful Ordering:

- **Ask for Modifications:** Don't hesitate to ask for modifications to your dish, such as dressing on the side, no added spices, or substitutions for trigger foods.
- **Control Portion Sizes:** Opt for smaller portions or consider splitting a dish with a dining companion to avoid overeating.

3. Be Conscious of Trigger Foods:

- **Identify Trigger Foods:** Be aware of your personal trigger foods, such as citrus, tomatoes, spicy dishes, and fatty or fried foods. Try to avoid or limit them.
- **Watch for Hidden Triggers:** Some sauces, dressings, or marinades may contain hidden triggers. Ask about ingredients or choose dishes with simple preparations.

4. Hydration and Timing:

- **Choose Water or Non-Citrus Beverages:** Opt for water, herbal tea, or non-citrus beverages instead of acidic or carbonated options.

- **Be Mindful of Timing:** Avoid eating too close to bedtime. Allow at least 2-3 hours between eating and lying down to minimize the risk of acid reflux.

5. Socializing Strategies:

- **Eat Slowly and Mindfully:** Take your time to chew thoroughly and enjoy your meal. Eating slowly can help prevent overeating and reduce the risk of heartburn.

- **Engage in Conversation:** Participate in conversations during meals to distract yourself from overeating and to promote mindful eating.

- **Select Appetizers Wisely:** Choose lighter appetizers or salads as a starter to help control overall calorie intake.

6. Dessert Decisions:

- **Opt for Low-Acid or GERD-Friendly Desserts:** Choose desserts with lower acidity, such as baked fruits, sorbet, or non-citrus options.
- **Share Desserts:** Consider sharing a dessert with others to satisfy your sweet tooth without consuming a large portion.

7. Planning Ahead:

- **Review Menus in Advance:** If possible, review the restaurant menu online before arriving to make informed and mindful choices.
- **Pack Antacids:** Carry antacids or medications prescribed by your healthcare professional in case of unexpected symptoms.

8. Communicate with Servers:

- **Inform Servers about Your Dietary Needs:** Let the server know about your dietary preferences and any restrictions related to

GERD. They can provide guidance and communicate your needs to the kitchen.

9. Alcohol Moderation:

- **Choose Low-Acid Options:** If you choose to drink alcohol, opt for low-acid options such as white wine or light beer. Avoid citrus-based cocktails.

- **Moderation is Key:** Limit alcohol intake, as excessive consumption can exacerbate GERD symptoms.

10. Plan for Success:

- **Bring GERD-Friendly Snacks:** If you're attending a social event, consider bringing GERD-friendly snacks to ensure you have options that align with your dietary needs.

11. Listen to Your Body:

- **Pay Attention to Signals:** Listen to your body and pay attention to how different foods affect you. If you start to feel discomfort, take a break from eating.

12. Relaxation Techniques:

- **Practice Relaxation Before Meals:** Engage in relaxation techniques such as deep breathing or mindfulness before meals to reduce stress, which can contribute to GERD symptoms.

CONCLUSION

Encouragement and Next Steps:

Embracing a GERD-friendly lifestyle is a positive and empowering choice that can significantly improve your overall well-being. By making thoughtful changes to your diet and lifestyle, you can manage GERD symptoms effectively and enjoy a healthier, more fulfilling life.

Embrace the Journey to Wellness:

1. **Mindful Eating:** Approach meals with mindfulness, savoring each bite and paying attention to your body's signals. Enjoying your food in a relaxed manner can contribute to better digestion.

2. **Stress Management:** Incorporate stress-reducing activities into your routine, such as yoga, meditation, or deep breathing exercises. Managing stress is crucial for minimizing GERD symptoms.

3. Stay Hydrated: Drinking plenty of water helps with digestion and can alleviate symptoms. Choose non-citrus, non-acidic beverages to stay hydrated throughout the day.

4. Regular Physical Activity: Engage in regular, gentle physical activity. Exercise can aid digestion and contribute to maintaining a healthy weight, which is beneficial for managing GERD.

5. Quality Sleep: Ensure you get adequate and quality sleep. Elevating your upper body slightly while sleeping may reduce nighttime symptoms.

www.ingramcontent.com/pod-product-compliance
Lightning Source LLC
Chambersburg PA
CBHW050844260726
48660CB00006B/2431